SANITARY COMMISSION.
(N.)

REPORT

OF A

COMMITTEE OF THE ASSOCIATE MEDICAL MEMBERS

OF THE

SANITARY COMMISSION

ON THE SUBJECT OF

SCURVY

WITH

SPECIAL REFERENCE TO PRACTICE IN THE ARMY AND NAVY.

WASHINGTON:
GOVERNMENT PRINTING OFFICE.
1862.

ON SCURVY.

Scurvy is a disease which, from whatever point it is regarded, cannot fail to attract the attention of the thoughtful military surgeon. Formerly its victims in armies and navies were to be counted by thousands annually, and if at the present time its ravages are not so extensive as a few years since, the fact that it is still not infrequently met with shows that either we are not cognizant of all its causes or that we ignorantly or wilfully allow those circumstances to exist by which it inevitably will be induced.

The subject is one also which ought, in many of its connections, to receive the earnest consideration of every military commander who has the good of his troops at heart. It lies with him to carry out those hygienic measures which his medical staff may recommend, and he ought to know that the occurrence of one single case of this disease in his command shows the existence of causes which will surely give rise to it in others, and in a short time render his force miserable, inefficient, and a burden to the public it was intended to serve. Scurvy is preëminently a preventable disease, and its existence in an army is *prima facie* evidence that the medical or military authorities have been neglectful of their duties.

It would be manifestly out of place in an essay of the purely practical character of this to enter at length into the history of the disease under consideration. It would appear, however, that it was not altogether unknown to the ancients, and that it was cured, as at present, by the use of fresh vegetable food.

Modern armies and navies from the year 1260, when it attacked the army of Louis IX in Egypt, have never been free from it the entire twelve months. During the seventeenth and eighteenth centuries, when so many naval expeditions of warfare and discovery were fitted out, whole crews were destroyed by it, and in the course of the same periods it more than decimated the armies of several European nations.

In more recent times, and notwithstanding the great advance which has been made in the knowledge of preventing and curing scurvy, it has not failed to take its victims by large numbers. Not to refer to other instances, it may be stated that our own armies have suffered greatly through its ravages. On one occasion, at Council Bluffs, in 1820, nearly the entire garrison was attacked, and many died. In Florida and in Mexico the efficiency of our forces was very materially lessened by its occurrence, and in Texas, New Mexico, and other frontier districts, cases of it have existed every year. In 1850 and 1851, it was very prevalent in New Mexico, and was in many instances extremely severe in its character.

The numerous emigrants to the west have been attacked with scurvy to a great extent. In 1848 and 1849 several overland parties *en route* to California and Oregon were almost destroyed by it, and in 1855 and 1856 the writer witnessed many cases among the settlers in Kansas.

In the Crimea, the English and French armies were afflicted with scurvy to an extent almost inconceivable at the present day. We shall have occasion hereafter to again advert to this circumstance. Let us take care that our own large army is kept free from this scourge

SYMPTOMS.—The symptoms of scurvy are generally sufficiently apparent to be recognised by the careful physician. The swollen and discolored gums, bleeding upon the slightest touch, the leaden hue of the features, the peculiarly offensive breath, the appearance of patches of extravasated blood, first upon the legs, but subsequently upon other parts of the body, the hardness and permanent state of contraction of the muscles, the stiffness of the joints, the re-opening of old ulcers and cicatrices, the re-solution of united fractures, the general œdema of the body, the diarrhœa and dysentery, and hæmorrhage from the mucous passages generally, the extreme mental depression and indisposition to any kind of exertion, are all often met with in one individual, and then present a picture which can scarcely lead to an error in diagnosis. There are cases, however, which cannot be so readily detected, because few of the prominent symptoms above mentioned are present. In such instances the existence of scurvy can generally be inferred with certainty from the existence of peculiar circumstances to which we shall hereafter direct attention.

The description of scurvy given by *Larrey is so graphic and truthful that we may be pardoned for reproducing it here. Speaking of the scurvy, as it appeared in the army of Egypt, he says:

"I have almost invariably remarked three different degrees in this scorbutic disease as in that which I had occasion to observe during my campaign in North America.

"In the first the soldier is distressed and prone to melancholy; he prefers the sitting or recumbent posture; he is

*Memoires de Chirurgie Militaire et Campagnes, Tome II, Paris, 1812, p. 272.

not disposed to be moved by those things which ordinarily excite his mind; the approach of the enemy, the various incidents of the camp, make no impression on him; he loses his appetite, sleep is painful, and is interrupted by disagreeable dreams; the countenance becomes pale, the eyes have a melancholy expression, and are surrounded by bluish circles; the gums are painful, pale, and bleed easily on the slightest pressure; heavy pains are felt in the lumbar region and in the limbs, especially the legs; respiration is difficult and the pulse is slow and irregular; the cutaneous transpiration is arrested and the skin becomes dry and rough, like that of a plucked fowl; the bowels become constipated; the urine is secreted in small quantity, and is loaded with earthy matters; the cutaneous veins are swollen, especially those of the groin; the patient experiences a feeling of lassitude in all his limbs, and walks with great difficulty.

"Wounds quickly change their character; suppuration diminishes and becomes sanguinollent; the lips of the wound are discolored; the granulations are feeble; they are bluish, painful, and bleed on the least touch. Cicatrices assume a peculiar appearance; they become discolored, ulcerate, and are liable to mortification. This first stage indicates the loss of tone, general debility, and a diminution of the vital principle.

"In the second stage, the symptoms become more intense; the feeling of prostration augments; the pains become more violent and are located especially in the head and kidneys; the patient falls into a state of stupor; he remains almost immovable in bed; his limbs are flexed and his whole body curved; his countenance and lips are livid; the white of the eyes changes to a leaden color; the breath becomes fetid, the gums ulcerated, and the teeth covered with black tartar. The respiration is now difficult and is accompanied with oppression and constriction of the chest; the cellular tissue of the legs becomes engorged, especially that which is interposed between the tendo achillis and the tibia, and the swelling extends very soon to the rest of the limbs. This engorgement has more hardness than simple œdema, the impression of the finger not remaining so long as in the latter case. Pressure causes pain; black spots are perceived over the malleoli and along the course of the tibia; they also appear about the same time on the face and on the shoulders. The constipation increases; the abdomen becomes tumefied; the patient experiences a very strong feeling of heat in the præcordial region and a dull heavy pain about the hypochondria. The pulse is accelerated; an accession of fever occurs towards evening; wakefulness—during which state the pains are aggravated—is very distressing to the patient. The gangrenous condition which is manifested in the wounds or cicatrices progresses. Hæmorrhage becomes more frequent; the blood is black, very liquid, and coagulates with difficulty. The callus of fractures softens; the fragments become disunited and a kind of caries attacks the broken extremities which become denuded of periosteum and sometimes enormously swollen.

"In this second stage, nature, endeavoring to conquer the obstacles which impede the exercise of the functions, redoubles her energy, and in order to reëstablish the equilibrium seeks to resume the forces she has lost; but it is ordinarily in vain, and an increased degree of asthenia very soon succeeds these reactions.

"The last stage of scurvy presents a most afflicting aspect. To the febrile paroxysms and the other symptoms I have described succeeds a general depression. The swelling of the feet and legs sensibly increases, and they become covered with black spots which, by their rapid communication with each other, give a character of sphacelus to the whole member.

* * * * * * * *

"I return to the other symptoms of this stage of scurvy. The tongue is covered with a viscous and brownish-colored coating; the ulceration of the gums extends deeply towards the alveoli and interior of the mouth, attacking the veil of the palate and even the palatine arch. The teeth become loosened, and their loss is often accompanied with hæmorrhage difficult to be arrested. The eyes have a pleading expression, and the eyelids are swollen and puffy; a cold sweat of a nauseous odor appears over the whole body but chiefly over the abdomen and extremities. It is this which gives so shining an appearance to the skin. The sphincters of the anus become relaxed and diarrhœa which often degenerates into a dysenteric and colliquative flux becomes established. The urine is passed with difficulty on account of the paralysis of the bladder which ensues. The catheter must then be frequently passed or even left in the bladder permanently. The difficulty of breathing and oppression become extreme, and severe fits of coughing often cause the viscid mucus expectorated to be tinged with blood of a black color and fetid odor. The pulse becomes weaker, wiry, and disappears insensibly. The forces of the individual are entirely extinguished and he has frequent attacks of syncope. The black spots which were at first simply ecchymoses assume the character of a true gangrene which destroys the organ it attacks. Dropsy appears, the vital functions cease, and the patient slowly but surely expires."

But, as we have already said, it is not to be supposed that

scurvy is always thus clearly manifested. Cases are frequently met with in which another disease seems to be present, but which is only a symptom of the scorbutic disorder. Or the scurvy may be so overshadowed by a coexistent affection as to render its presence more a matter of inference than of actual proof. We propose to devote a short space to the consideration of these complications.

Scurvy is frequently met with associated with dysentery and typhus and typhoid fevers. We have had many examples of these combinations under our charge. Dr. Tholozan, in a paper read before the French Academy of Medicine, thus alludes to them :

"Dysentery, scorbutus, and typhus, such as we know them by classical description, consist of groups of morbid phenomena perfectly distinct from each other. When these affections are met with singly in an uncomplicated state, it is easy to recognise them, and no observer will be deceived by them. But when the diseases are mingled one with the other, or, as sometimes happens, when all three are conjoined, forming, as has been so often observed in armies, compound diseases of mixed character of special types, the pathological problem becomes complicated. Dysentery presents the characteristics of scorbutus, scorbutus is attended with delirium, as is typhus, or rather dysenteric fluxes carry off the patient, and those affected with typhus, have dysentery and become scorbutic. Examples of these mixtures are not rare, for almost all serious cases are thus complicated. Such at least was my experience during the winter of 1854–'55, at Constantinople."

*Pincoffs also points out the frequency with which scurvy was conjoined with other diseases during the Crimean war. He says :

*Experiences of a civilian in eastern military hospitals, &c.

"Typhus was at that time [the winter of 1854–'55,] raging fiercely, and I am convinced that if not its main cause, certainly the cause of its great mortality was the scurvy. Of twenty patients admitted during that period eighteen were usually more or less scorbutic; eight perhaps would be so deeply affected (as indicated by sloughing ulcers, gangrene of the mouth, general dropsy, and chronic diarrhœa) as to render recovery impossible."

He also gives it as his opinion that of the 23,587 cases of diseases of the stomach and bowels, 10,970 cases of fevers, and 2,023 of frost-bites, which occurred, the great majority were scorbutic.

*Macleod also refers to the fact, that among the troops serving in the Crimea, scurvy was not usually discernible by the ordinary signs, by reason of its being so frequently masked behind some other ailment.

In the official reports made to the British government by the medical officers, the same facts are asserted. Thus it is said : †

"From the details now submitted, it will be readily understood that scurvy was an affection of some importance at one period in the army. It is to be observed, however, that the returns convey but a faint conception of the disastrous part which it acted among the troops; for although it was only in comparatively rare instances that it presented itself in well defined forms, and as an independent affection, yet the prevalence of scorbutic taint was wide-spread, and in a vast proportion of cases, evident indications of it existed as a complication of other diseases, fever and affec-

* Notes on the Surgery of the War in the Crimea. London: 1858, p. 69.

† Medical and Surgical History of the British Army which served in Turkey and the Crimea, &c., vol. 2, p. 171.

tions of the bowels. Indeed, it may be stated, that during the first six months of the siege, all morbid actions in the older residents were more or less distinctly marked by scorbutic symptoms; and the fact is constantly commented upon by medical officers. Thus, Dr. Marlow, 28th regiment, remarks: 'although there are apparently few cases of pure scurvy marked in the return, nearly every admission into hospital exhibited unequivocal signs of the scorbutic taint.' "

To return to the French authorities, we find that Baudens* also points out that, "scorbutus prevailed under an epidemic form and was rarely witnessed without being complicated with diarrhœa, intermittent and remittent fever, bronchitis, pneumonia, &c. These complications were the most direct causes of the mortality which scurvy produced."

Scrive† states that "at the end of February more than three thousand cases of scurvy in which the disease was well marked existed. Some patients had only scurvy; in others it was associated with diarrhœa, dysentery, and typhus or typhoid affections, above all with frost-bites, to which it greatly increased the liability. These combinations were all-powerful; the sick were unable to resist them, and succumbed to swell the daily-augmenting record of our mortality."

During the service of the writer in New Mexico and Kansas, many cases of scurvy were witnessed which were more or less marked by some more prominent affection. Diarrhœa and dysentery, were frequent complications, and were often the only evidences of a scorbutic taint, except

* La Guerre Crimée, &c. Paris, 1858, p. 219.

†Relation Medico Chirurgicale de la Campagne d'Orient. Paris, 1857, p. 389.

sometimes the presence of very small ecchymoses on the legs scarcely distinguishable from flea-bites. These latter were not always to be detected, and yet there could be no doubt in regard to the scorbutic character of the disease, for it always readily yielded to anti-scorbutic treatment, and as obstinately resisted that directed against the obvious characteristics.

But perhaps the most common symptom of scurvy, liable to lead to an erroneous diagnosis which the writer has witnessed, was one similating what ordinarily passes under the name of chronic rheumatism. This consisted of very severe pains in the muscles of the legs and back, increasing in severity towards evening. The appearance of the skin was not in the least altered for some time, neither was there any particular tenderness of the gums. The muscles were not permanently contracted nor abnormally hard. The progress of the disease was in many of these cases arrested at this point by appropriate treatment, but in others it passed on to well-developed scurvy. There is, we think, but little doubt that many of the cases designated in the medical reports as chronic rheumatism are in reality of a scorbutic nature. In the official work* from which we have already quoted, mention is thus made in regard to the point in question:

"One of the most constant precursory symptoms of scurvy was an obscure form of muscular rheumatism. The individual complained of pains in his legs of an aching character, and his movements were tedious and painful; there was in these cases no articular inflammation observed, and though the feet and legs were generally œdematous, there was little enlargement of the ankle joints; the affec-

* Medical and Surgical History of the British Army, &c., &c., p. 175.

tion has probably been in some instances mistaken for rheumatism and perhaps treated in the ordinary manner, but it was merely one of the signs of general cachexia, and advantageously treated by a return to the comforts of ordinary life.

Hemeralopia and nyctalopia, which are not infrequently met with among soldiers and sailors, are undoubtedly often due to a scorbutic taint. Dr. Coale,* U. S. Navy, noticed several cases of the latter in the scurvy which occurred on board the frigate Columbia in 1838–'39 and '40. Dr. Foltz† witnessed several cases of both these singular affections as accompaniments to the scurvy, which attacked the crew of the United States frigate Raritan in 1846.

In the Crimean war hemeralopia, though not adverted to in the official reports from which we have already quoted, was, according to Macleod,‡ a common attendant on scurvy as it appeared among the British troops.

The writer has seen but two cases of either affection which were of undoubted scorbutic character. Both of these were hemeralopia or day blindness, and occurred in New Mexico. The blindness was almost complete on bright clear days. As evening approached the patients began to see with more distinctness, and at dusk possessed nearly the natural powers of vision.

We must not forget to allude to the influence of the scorbutic diathesis in modifying the character of wounds, in causing gangrene, in the production of bed-sores, in preventing the reunion of fractured bones, &c., we cannot, however, do more than simply call attention to these complications.

*American Journal of the Medical Sciences, vol. III, p. 68.
†American Journal of the Medical Sciences, vol. XV, p. 38.
‡Op. Cit. p. 71.

We have pointed out, at some length, associations of scurvy with other disorders, because we are satisfied from much observation that a powerful cause of these diseases, the scorbutic condition of the system is frequently overlooked, both in diagnosis and treatment. The military medical officer cannot be too circumspect in his examination of patients who are subjected to conditions favorable to the development of scurvy. He will frequently find, by careful observation, that his numerous cases of typhoid fever, diarrhœa, dysentery, rheumatism, frost-bites, &c., are in great part due to that depraved state of the blood which is the essential characteristic of scurvy, even though many prominent symptoms of the latter disease be absent, and he will find that by enforcing proper sanitary and medicinal treatment, the diseases which have resisted all his routine measures will be driven out, or, what is infinitely better, entirely prevented.

Pathology.—It would not comport with the purely practical character of this memoir to dwell to any extent upon the pathology of scurvy. In order, however, to inculcate a clear idea of the prophylaxis and treatment it will be necessary to bring some of the more prominent points of this portion of the subject before the reader.

We naturally look in the first place to the state of the blood, and we find a very decided change from the normal condition of this fluid. We shall give an abstract only of our own researches on this point.

1st. The amount of *water* is increased and the total amount of *solid matter* diminished.

2d. The *fibrin* is augmented in quantity.

3d. There is a decided diminuation in the amount of *blood corpuscles.*

4th. The *albumen* is also diminished in quantity.

5th. The amount of *inorganic constituents* is very materially lessened, principally through the diminution in the quantity of *potash*, *lime*, and *iron* normally present in the blood.

These are the chief alterations which (as several analyses of the blood have enabled us to ascertain) attend the presence of scurvy.

It is scarcely reasonable to hold the opinion that any one of these alterations in the normal character of the blood is the immediate *cause* of the scorbutic diathesis. Garrod believes that a deficiency of potash in the system is the cause of scurvy. We confess to having once held a similar opinion, but more extensive observation has satisfied us of its incorrectness. The fact, that under the influence of potash scurvy disappears, is no valid argument in support of the theory in question, for, as we have ascertained, iron also effects a cure and with as much rapidity as potash. No doubt the deficiency of potash is an important point in the pathology of the disease, but it is to all the alterations in the normal constitution of the blood that we are to look for the immediate cause of the scorbutic diathesis.

We have seen that it is more than probable the immediate or essential cause of scruvy is a morbid alteration in the constitution of the blood. We come, in the next place, to consider the predisposing or exciting cause.

It was formerly held that the long-continued use of salt food was the chief cause of the development of scurvy. There was apparently just ground for this opinion, for the disease was observed chiefly among those who for long periods were subjected to this kind of diet. It is now, however, very well established that the use of salt food alone will not ordinarily excite the disease. Along with the restriction to this species of nutriment we have various other coexisting circumstances which have fully as much if not more power in giving rise to the scorbutic diathesis.

The causes of scurvy may very properly be considered under three heads. The *physical*, the *moral*, and the *dietic*.

Physical causes.—Darkness and *cold* are important agents in causing scurvy. Arctic voyagers have had abundant opportunity for noticing their influence. During the arctic winter it has been uniformly the case that scurvy prevailed more extensively than during the summer, although there was no difference in the character of the food. Dr. I. I. Hayes has informed the writer that there can be no doubt on this point. Of themselves, however, they are not sufficient, for during the recent voyage of this eminent traveller and discoverer, scurvy was entirely prevented by the excellent hygienic measures he adopted, and to which we shall soon have occasion to allude.

Moisture is also a powerful cause of scurvy. This was very evident in the Crimea, where the men of the allied army were exposed in the trenches and even in their tents and huts to an excessive amount of moisture for a long period.

Impure air is another influential physical cause of scurvy. Dr. Hayes ascribes his immunity from scurvy chiefly to the excellent system of ventilation he adopted. In the United States Navy it has frequently been noticed that scurvy was much more violent in those ships in which little attention was given to renewing the atmosphere, than in those where good ventilation was insisted upon. We have several times had occasion to notice the appearance of this disease among troops crowded into small barracks, whilst those who had plenty of room escaped, though the other conditions were the same. In New Mexico, soldiers were often packed at night in two or three tiers of beds, with two in a bed. There can be no doubt as to the state of the atmosphere by morning, and its influence in causing scurvy was well marked.

It often happens that the physical conditions we have mentioned occur together. Dr. Opitz,* in an excellent monograph, shows that cold, humidity, and bad air were the chief if not the only causes of the epidemic of scurvy which attacked the Austrian garrison at Ranstatt in 1852. Out of 4,300 men, 610 had scurvy. The unfavorable state of the atmosphere, moisture combined with cold, and the oppressive and miasmatic character of the air in the over-crowded locality of the barracks, are the causes to which Opitz mainly ascribes the epidemic.

Insufficient exercise on the one hand and *excessive physical exertion* on the other, are among the exciting causes of scurvy. The influence of the former has been perceived among the arctic explorers, and the over-worked soldiers of the allied army afforded marked examples of the power of the latter cause.

The *moral causes* of scurvy, though perhaps not so apparent in their influence as those we have mentioned, are, nevertheless, of very considerable importance.

Nostalgia is a common exciting cause of scurvy. To this, and the *despondency of mind* which attends it, the attacks of scurvy which have proved so fatal to arctic adventurers owe much of their violence. So well is *mental depression* recognised as a cause of the disease in question, that arctic navigators have taken every means in their power to guard against it.

* Ueber Skorbut: Vierteljahrschrift für die praktische Heil Kunde, Band 69, 1861, p. 108.

We are convinced that many cases of scurvy occurring among overland emigrants to Oregon and California are due to despondency and anxiety. During periods of weary inaction, or the depression of mind produced by disaster and defeat, scurvy has always been more persistent and violent in armies and fleets.

Dietetic causes.—Undoubtedly the most efficient agents in the causation of scurvy are those arising from the long-continued use of food deficient in these substances which the organism requires for its perfect nutrition, or else of too unvarying a character.

For a long time it was supposed that scurvy was due to the continued ingestion of *salt meat.* It is doubtful, however, that such is the case. It is not so much the use of salt food as it is the deprivation of succulent vegetable food, which induces scurvy. Dr. Hayes has, however, recently informed the writer that he thinks the immunity of his command from scurvy was, in great part, due to the fact that the men had such an abundance of fresh reindeer meat that they did not have to resort at all to the salt provisions. There are, nevertheless, many examples on record of scurvy appearing when fresh meat has formed the staple article of diet, and we have ourselves witnessed many cases of the disease among troops who had fresh meat four days out of the seven as a part of their ration, and who had it the other three from game which they procured for themselves. It must not be forgotten, also, that Dr. Hayes had an abundance of anti-scorbutics, of which the men had an ample allowance, and that he employed every other means to prevent the disease.

The *deprivation of fresh vegetable food* is undoubtedly a powerful cause of scurvy. It is very rare that this disease makes its appearance where an abundance of such food can be obtained. It is not, however, to be inferred that scurvy does not occasionally appear among people who eat a great deal of fresh vegetable food. In such cases the moral and physical causes we have mentioned are so strong as to overcome every resistance. Dr. Pincoffs, in the work from which we have quoted, says that "Turks who eat but little meat and a great deal of fruit suffered greatly with scurvy. Dr. Leudersdoff, who had charge of a Turkish hospital during the Crimean war, had sixty, of his beds filled with scorbutic cases, and the same, he says, was the case with all the hospitals, large and small, at Eupatoria. There are many examples on record of the disease appearing when fresh vegetables were supplied in abundance."

Perhaps a more influential cause than a salt-meat diet or the mere deprivation of fresh vegetable food, is found in the *sameness of diet* to which soldiers and sailors are so frequently subjected.

The following extract from a work* we have already quoted from, places the whole subject of food as a cause of scurvy in its true position :

"It has hitherto been too constantly supposed, at least by the community in general, that scurvy is mainly, if not altogether, to be attributed to the use of salt provisions, and that it is little to be apprehended unless these form a large proportion of the daily food; but the fact is, paradoxical as it may appear, that it would be extremely difficult to prove that scurvy has any other closer connection with the use of salt meat than of fresh meat, for the disease is observed not alone when salt provisions constitute the

* Medical and Surgical History of the British Army, which served in Turkey and the Crimea, &c., vol. II, p. 179.

food, but when the diet is composed exclusively of fresh provisions. Thus, after the campaign of 1848–'49, (which terminated in the annexation of the Punjaub,) the agricultural operations of a portion of that province were for a season interrupted, and the troops, which were placed in occupation, suffered accordingly from the want of fresh vegetables. They were, nevertheless, supplied with abundance of fresh meat and bread of excellent quality, and yet, in the 24th regiment, the annual return recorded the occurrence of several cases of scurvy. The disease also showed itself in other corps to such a degree, that it was found necessary to send to a great distance, and at considerable expense, for supplies of potatoes. The principal medical officer, pending their arrival in sufficient abundance, recommending them to be used as a salad, dressed with vinegar, in order to procure their full curative effects.

"Again, for some years after the different stations for troops were formed in the Himalaya mountains, fresh vegetables, from the position of these stations, were not procurable in sufficient quantity, while at a subsequent date the supplies were interrupted by the breaking out of the Sutlej war; but though the soldier was provided with good fresh meat and bread, yet scurvy was not only present but attended with its full share of mortality, both among men and women; and it became necessary to relieve corps at short intervals, after they had, in some degree, recovered from the relaxation of long-continued residence in the hot climate of the plains, and before they had too deeply acquired the scorbutic taint in the hills. In this instance the direct causes of dysentery were present—dense fogs, periodic rains, cold winds, and elevated locality; and scurvy appeared in association with dysentery; and it was here that the term scorbutic dysentery was first recognised, we believe, in a general sense, as one of proper application.

"Sir John Hall, speaking of the causes of scurvy, observes 'much stress has been laid on the use of salt meat in producing scurvy; my own opinion is, that other agencies were in operation to induce the depression of the vital powers, and generate the cachectic condition which the men fell into; for I have seen as much scurvy at the Cape, in the campaign of 1846–'47, as occurred in the Crimea; and at the Cape no salt meat was consumed by a man in the field. Fatigue, wet, cold, and exposure, with sameness of diet,' he adds, 'will produce scurvy without salt meat. At the Cape, rice was an integral portion of the men's rations during the whole campaign; and if this article had been issued in December and January, 1854–'55, in the Crimea, the results would have been nearly the same.'

"Dr. Crawford refering to the appearance of scurvy in the 18th regiment during the last winter in the Crimea, offers the following remarks in illustration of the causes of scurvy, and the nature of their action:

"'When men are placed for any length of time on a particular diet, without the opportunity of augmenting it by the addition of articles which instinct teaches them to seek out, a nice adjustment of the proportion which the various nutritious principles should be as to each other, and to the circumstances in which the individuals so dieted are placed, is essential to health. The substitution of one class of nutritious elements for another, or the absence of a due proportion of either, will soon show itself. An instance of this sort occurred during the second Burmese war. A detachment of Europeans stationed at Meanday, were dieted for several months on fresh beef, in unlimited quantities, biscuit, with the usual allowance of rum and rice, but they were not supplied with fresh vegetables, or any substitute for them. At first the men looked robust and healthy, but after the lapse of three months, scurvy made its appearance; spongy gums, purple blotches on the extremities, hemorrhagic dysentery and profuse discharges of blood from the stomach and bowels, (during the hot stage of intermittent fevers then prevalent,) marked the outset of the disease. Lime-juice was procured and issued freely, and the scurvy rapidly abated. Lime-juice or the salts rich in potass,' he continues, 'will generally check scurvy under such circumstances; and', 'he adds, it is scarcely necessary to remark that the nitrogenous or albuminous elements were superabundant in this case.'"

The report then goes on to state:

"As military experience has thus shown that scurvy under certain circumstances attends upon the use of exclusively fresh provisions, it must be conceded that salt food has no peculiar, or, at least, exclusive connection with the disease; and that if the affection has more often accompanied its use, it is only because there is some coöperating agency frequently associated with the consumption of salt food which can have no place when fresh provisions constitute the diet, except under very unusual or artificial conditions of life. This agency is no other than want of variety of food—sameness in diet; and if we may consider the effect of it acting in connection with the use of fresh food, under unusual conditions of life, to be illustrated by the facts above mentioned, its consequences under artificial conditions of life, the work of our own creation, have perhaps been abundantly testified in the history of our jails, workhouses, and, it may be, also, to some extent, of our schools and factories.

"The want of variety in food constitutes the true cause of scurvy; but the diversity essential to its prevention or cure does not consist simply in the use of animal and vegetable food, but of animal food, with vegetable food of *varied properties.* We have already seen that scurvy, and its associated affections, may appear under the exclusive use of fresh meat and bread, but we are not aware that the disease has ever been observed when the diet was composed of meat and of vegetables of various kinds in due proportion."

But we are satisfied that neither the physical, the moral, nor the dietetic causes of scurvy are of themselves alone sufficient to produce the disease. It is only when all three are conjoined that scurvy makes its appearance. Perhaps the most influential cause is the want of variation in the diet, so strongly insisted upon in the foregoing extracts; but this of itself will not give rise to scurvy, otherwise we should see the Indians of our western prairies constantly afflicted with it, and the Esquimaux would never be free from the scorbutic diathesis. When we have insufficient food conjoined with mental depression and exposure to wet and cold, we have scurvy, and not otherwise.

It is extremely important not to forget this fact. It is too much the custom in the army to lay all the stress upon faulty diet, and to entirely ignore the physical and moral causes of scurvy. The medical officer should therefore be on his guard against all these influences. He can do much to counteract their power.

Prevention of scurvy.—When we know the causes of a disease we can do much towards preventing it. When scurvy occurs, some one is to blame; for its causes are altogether under our control. As the causes of scurvy are physical, moral, and dietetic, our measures of prevention come under the same heads.

Physical means of prevention.—First among them is the adoption of measures to secure a due allowance of pure air. This can readily be done in barracks by giving to each soldier at least six hundred cubic feet of space, and opening the window (where other means of ventilation are not provided) so as to allow of the free admission of the external air and the exit of that which has become impure. Soldiers, like civilians, have too great a horror of a draft of air, and positive orders and constant watching will be necessary to make them attend to this point.

In camp, the tents should not be placed too close together; should not be overcrowded, and should be struck every clear day, and the bedding, &c., thoroughly aired. At least once a week the tents should be moved a few feet so as to cover fresh ground.

In addition, a thorough state of police should be kept up. In one camp which the writer has recently visited as inspecting officer, the filth which had accumulated for six weeks was shoveled into the middle of the streets so as to form high ridges, and then left to decompose. Could anything be more disgusting?

Exposure to cold and wet cannot always in a military life be avoided; much may be done, however, by warm and impervious clothing to lessen their influence.

Moderate bodily exercise should always be insisted on. It is one of the best preventives of scurvy. Armstrong* states that the men of the Investigator were required to

* Observations on Naval Hygiene and Scurvy.

take five hours' exercise every day. Dr. Hayes, also, always made a point of insisting on a due amount of exercise being taken by each man of his command. We believe that to this action, and the thorough means he took to provide for ventilation, are in the main to be ascribed the freedom of his party from scurvy.

Immoderate bodily exertion, when required on the part of the soldiers by military necessity, must, of course, be submitted to. But there are times when it can be avoided. A good commander will never unnecessarily fatigue his men. Drills, or fatigue duty, before breakfast can almost always be deprived of their bad effects by serving out hot coffee to the men.

Moral means of prevention.—Much may be done to induce cheerfulness in an army. Games of various kinds, especially such as require exercise in the open air, should be encouraged. Sir Edward Parry, it is said, prevented scurvy in his command by using every means in his power to cause cheerful feeling to predominate. Books of a light character are useful agents towards this end. Theatres should likewise be encouraged. The regimental bands, however, are the most important means for conducing to cheerfulness in a command. Their usefulness in this respect cannot be overestimated, and it is to be hoped they will not be abolished. We have never seen an intelligent soldier who did not take pleasure in the music the bands afforded.

Dietetic means of prevention.—These means have always been held in high repute. When properly used they may be said to be infallible. For a great many years *lime-juice* has been regarded as the most valuable agent we possess for preventing scurvy. Since its use by the Dutch, in the early part of the sixteenth century, it has not lost in the estimation of the civilized world, and for many years has formed a component part of the ration of seamen so situated as to be liable to scurvy. In the English navy, lime-juice is issued when the men have been for fourteen days on salt-meat diet. By this one article scurvy has been almost eradicated from modern navies. Citric acid is not a substitute, it being almost entirely inert as we have found by experience.

It can scarcely be said that pure vegetable acids are anti-scorbutics. Vinegar cannot, therefore, be elevated to this rank. The lime-juice doubtless owes its valuable properties to the fact that it contains supercitrate of potassa.

We have already alluded to the efficacy of potash as an anti-scorbutic. In a paper published in the American Journal of the Medical Sciences for ——— we gave the results of our experience up to that time with potash in this connection. Since then we have had abundant opportunity of using it, and have seen nothing to cause us to modify the opinion then expressed of its great value. As a prophylactic of scurvy we regard it as invaluable. At Cebolletta, in New Mexico, where the writer was stationed several years, the men of the garrison never had scurvy originating in them at that place, though it prevailed very extensively at other ports in the territory. Upon analyzing the water in use it was found to contain a large proportion of potash, and to this fact the immunity from scurvy was attributed.

The bitartrate is perhaps the best form in which to employ potash as an anti-scorbutic. It is more easily preserved and transported than lime-juice, and is, moreover, cheaper. An ounce of it taken daily when the men are so situated as to render them liable to scurvy, would, we are confident, entirely prevent it. Dissolved as far as possible in water, with a little sugar added, it makes a very pleasant drink.

The efficacy of potash is inferentially very strongly supported by the fact that those vegetables which are most prized as anti-scorbutics contain it in larger quantity. Thus, besides the lime-juice, in which it exists as an acid salt, we find that *potatoes*, which are almost as efficacious, contain it in large quantities. In New Mexico, when the winter had passed, we found the best results were obtained from the use as a salad or greens of the *lambs' quarter*, *(chenopodium album,)* one of the first of the spring plants. The men devoured it with the greatest avidity. Upon analysis of the expressed juice we found it to abound in potash.

The *sorrel*, *(rumex acetosella,)* which has likewise proved of the greatest value as an anti-scorbutic, owes its power to the acid salt, the binoxalate of potassa, which it contains. Both these plants are found throughout the United States.

Pickles and *sauer kraut* are also valuable anti-scorbutics, though not to be compared with those named.

The French in the Crimea found great benefit from the use of the *dandelion*, *(leontodon taraxacum,)* which was largely gathered by the men, and which they ate with vinegar.

We might mention many other special anti-scorbutics, but we think enough has been said to direct attention to those which are most valuable. Almost any succulent vegetable will give such a variety to the ordinary diet of the soldier as to prevent the occurrence of scurvy. If our army should always get the full ration, (which is scarcely to be expected,) there would not be much probability of this disease making its appearance among our soldiers. Congress did a wise act in adding potatoes to the ration.

Treatment of scurvy.—Scarcely anything remains to be said under this head. The general treatment is that which we have indicated as best adapted to prevent the occurrence of scurvy. The special treatment must be directed to such prominent symptoms as particularly claim attention. The measures to be adopted are, however, at most merely adjuvants to those physical, moral, and dietetic means which we have already insisted upon, and which will of themselves eventually relieve any local manifestations of the disease. Swollen and spongy gums may, however, be washed with a solution of tannin or a dilute solution of persulphate of iron. Ulcers are to be treated according to the general principles applicable ; weak astringent or gently stimulating applications being generally the best.

Stiff joints are to be rubbed with a stimulating liniment and subjected frequently to passive motion. Should false anchylosis have occurred, the limb is to be forcibly extended and fixed by mechanical means. We have frequently succeeded in restoring complete motion under such circumstances by this measure.

A tonic course of treatment has been recommended in scurvy. We scarcely think it frequently necessary. *Iron*, however, is always beneficial and deserves to rank high as a remedy for scurvy. We have had no experience with it as a prophylactic, but as an antidote to the scorbutic diathesis it is very valuable. We have usually preferred the tincture of the chloride in doses of thirty drops three times a day. The beneficial effect soon becomes well marked.

Bathing frequently is also a valuable adjuvant. The bath should be tepid so as neither to exhaust or depress the vital powers.

In conclusion, we have only to repeat what we have already said, that scurvy is a pre-eminently preventable disease. A case of scurvy in a camp or garrison is a reproach to some one. Let the members of our profession who are charged with the medical care of our sick soldiers see to it that the reproach does not rest with them.

WILLIAM A. HAMMOND,
Chairman.
JOSEPH CARSON, M. D.
EDWARD HARTSHORNE, M. D.
WALTER F. ATLEE, M. D.
S. WEIR MITCHEL, M. D.

SANITARY COMMISSION.

(**N.**)

www.ingramcontent.com/pod-product-compliance
Lightning Source LLC
LaVergne TN
LVHW011133110826
845150LV00008B/2316

* 9 7 8 1 4 1 8 1 9 4 3 3 8 *